"Why do I need to get a shot?"

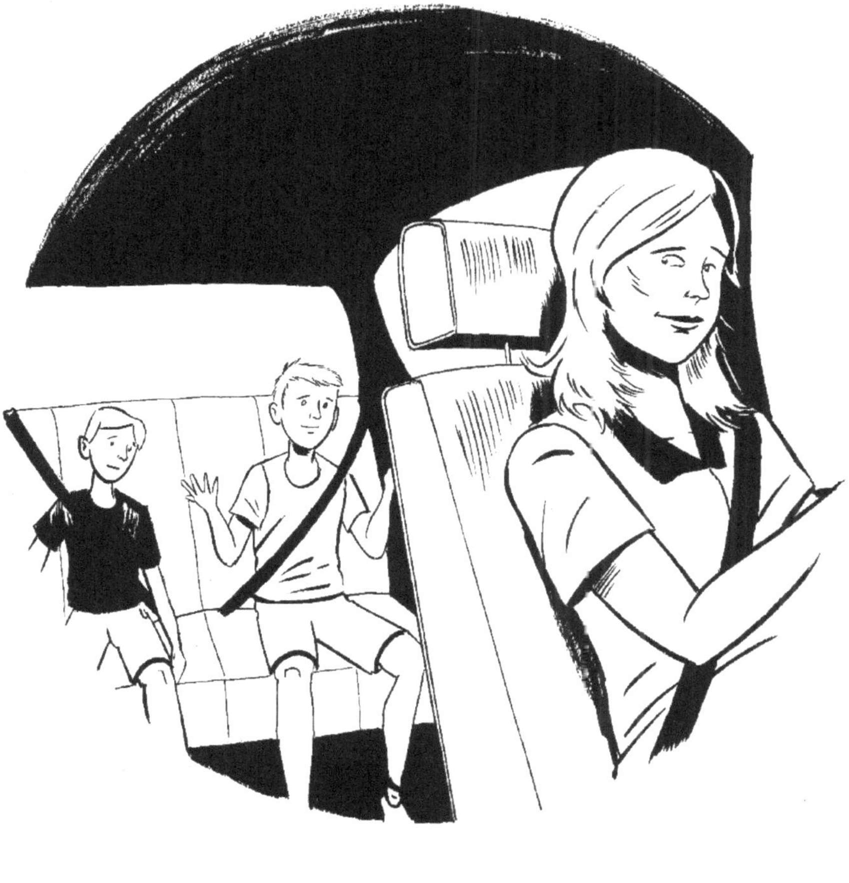

ISBN-10: 1535182539
ISBN-13: 978-1535182539

DEDICATION

This book is dedicated to the glittering Everlee Stevenson; whose strength, perseverance, and exuberant joy render her family forever grateful.

~~~~~~~~~~~~~~~~~~~~~~~~~~

This fictional story and coloring book is about two brothers who are going to the doctor for routine check ups and to receive their booster vaccinations. The intended message is to inform children and families about the necessity of vaccination, while addressing ways to cope with the stress involve with receiving booster shots.

I lagged and dawdled as I walked toward the car,

following my Mom's shadow, with my

brother not back far...

On our way to the doctor, I knew we would go.

My Mom started the car with the two of us in
tow.

"But why must we go today?" my voice rang with
fear,

"neither of us are sick, so why not just stay
here?"

"It is true, you're both healthy," she responded

with cheer,

Then she revved up her engine and continued to
steer.

"Your appointments are for 'well checks,' and there's no reason to whine,

or fuss, or fight, or worry; your health is surely fine."

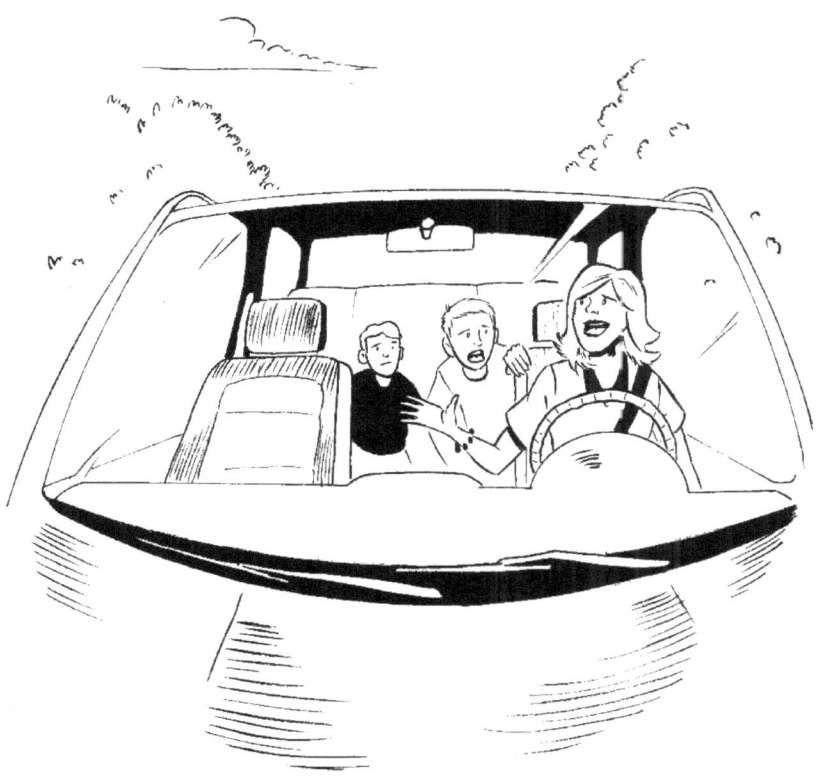

"What will the doctor check?" I asked. "My heart? My lungs? My weight?

And what about the duck-walk-test? Is that to check my gait?"

"That is all true!" she sounded amused, "the doctor will check you out,

to make sure you're growing healthy, from your feet up to your snout."

"But will we have to get shots today?" my brother whimpered with regret.

"Of course you'll receive vaccinations," she replied, "but there's no reason to fret."

My smile bent into a grimace, and my brother let out a "yelp!"

"I hate needles!" he fiercely shrieked, and I certainly was no help.

"WHAT?" "NO!" I screeched loudly, the fear was ringing from my voice,

"I will not go! I will not go!" I said....as if I had a choice.

"Please keep calm," my Mom replied as she rolled into the lot,

"There's no reason to be fearful kids, you know, it's just a shot."

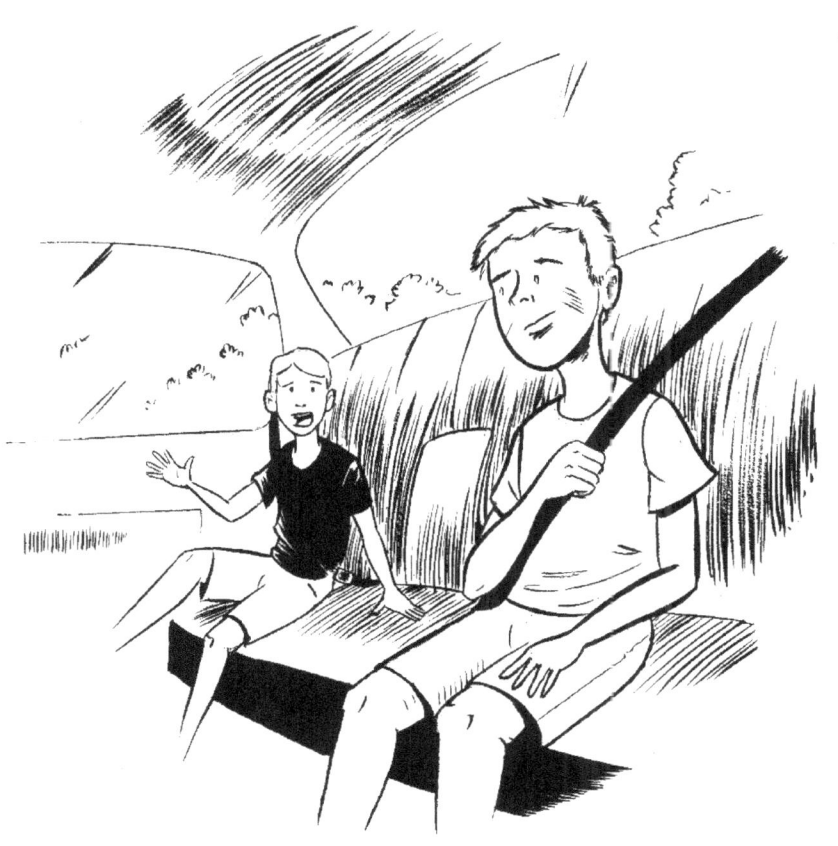

The nurse smiled at our sad faces as she checked our ears and eyes.

"You both seem very healthy!" she smiled. We could barely control our cries.

"Welcome kids! Lets check you out!" entered cheerful Dr. McCay.

"We'll look and listen from head to toe, and then we'll send you on your way."

My brother and I were courteous as Dr. McCay went about his work,

"Your lungs are clear, your heart tick-tocks, and your reflexes rightly jerk."

He raised his light up to my mouth, "Ah, quite a healthy throat and nose,"

He checked my tummy, bones, and muscles; then told me to wiggle my toes.

He finished up our check ups, and said, "You are both quite healthy and fit!

There is just one more thing to do to keep you from getting sick.

The nurse will be back shortly, to bring in the vaccines you will need."

With this I started whimpering, and my brother began to plead.

"Oh boys, what could be wrong?   What is with all this fright?

Vaccines are just a form of medicine that will help to keep you feeling right."

"But I hate needles, it hurts so much, and it makes me sore for days!

I'll wash my hands! I'll brush my teeth!" I pleaded, "Isn't there any other way?"

"I understand you're scared, but vaccines are designed to protect.

So that when dangerous germs loom in the air they may have less effect."

"What are these diseases?" I asked. "Well, there is pox, and mumps, and flu,

Polio, measles, and whooping cough, just to name a few.

You see, the medicine in these shots helps for your immune system to advance,

to build your bodies defenses so these diseases may have less of a chance."

I listened to Dr. McCay, and then asked something I have always wanted to know,

"Some of my friends don't get these vaccines, why do I have to though?"

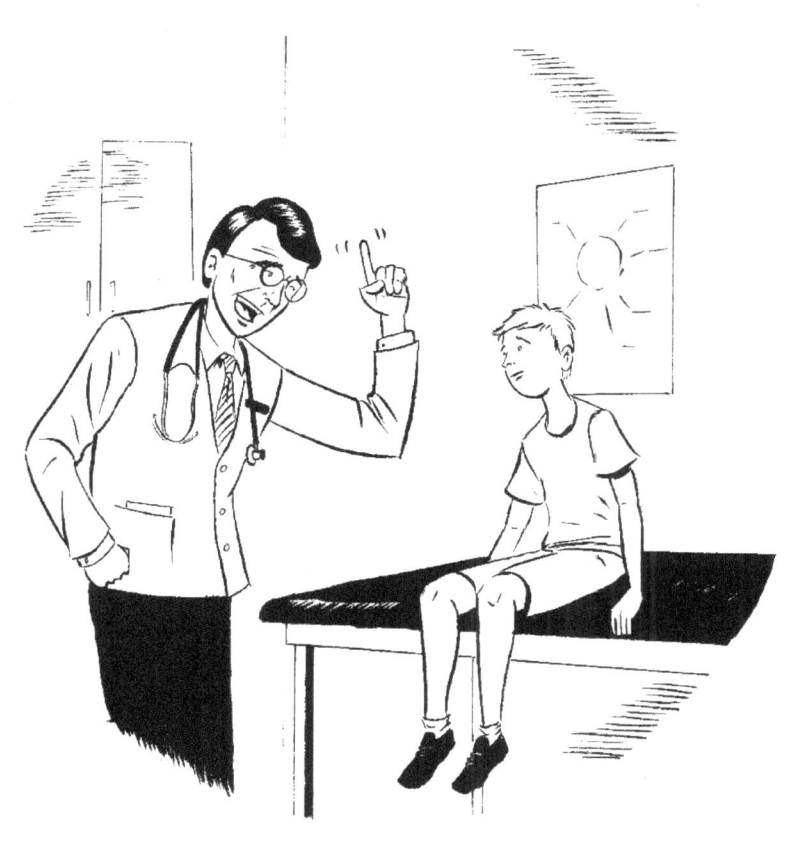

"I understand your question, and I am happy to explain;

when kids don't get vaccines, these diseases could cause serious pain."

"There are some kids who aren't able to receive vaccines, and there are some who simply choose,

But we know that being protected, is too important to refuse.

Because contact between people is how these diseases tend to spread,

And when fewer people are protected, the chances of getting sick may rise instead."

"I get it," my brother nodded, "I guess the shot is worth a little pain."

I agreed, "It sounds like protection from disease is quite a lot to gain."

Then I watched the needle poke my skin and leave a small red spot,

It was over before I knew it, Dr. McCay had helped a lot.

Our Mom thanked them for the check up, and we walked back through the door.

We were happy to be healthier now, than we were even before.

Next time we go to the doctor I will remember what I have been taught,

That protection from disease is worth a little shot.

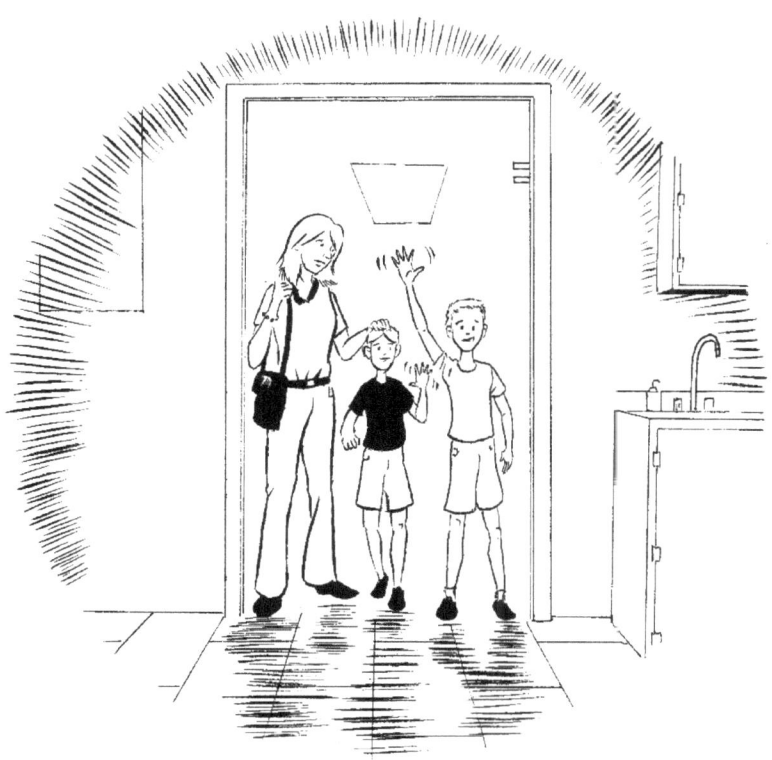

Now is it your turn to *share* your story:

Who are the people in your family? Draw a picture of your family.

What does is mean to be *strong* and *healthy?*

Draw a picture of your strong and healthy self.

Heroes are people who you admire.

Who are your heroes? What do your heroes look like? Draw a picture of your heroes.

Doctors can be heroes who can help to keep your family *strong* and *safe* by giving shots.

What does your strong face look like?

What *worries* do you have about getting shots at the doctor?

What does your worried face look like?

You are very *brave*.

It is important to be brave when facing things that make you feel afraid. What does your brave face look like?

Keeping yourself *healthy* is important.

What do you do to stay healthy? Washing your hands, eating healthy, getting enough sleep, exercising, and getting your vaccinations at the doctor are all great ways to stay healthy. Draw a picture of all the things you do to stay healthy.

Being healthy is *fun*!

When you are healthy you have energy for the things that you enjoy. What do you like to do when you are healthy? Draw a picture of these fun things.

Thank you for reading this story, and for sharing your own colorful story of good health!

Everlee's story:

When Everlee was only a few weeks old she was exposed to Pertussis (a.k.a. whooping cough). Her illness was very serious and she had to spend several weeks in the hospital. Thankfully, there is a vaccine called the "DTaP" that protects children against pertussis and other diseases. Everlee was too young to receive this vaccine when she got sick.

Everlee fought hard against this disease and eventually she got better. Her story is important to share because when children don't get vaccines, these serious diseases can spread to infants and other vulnerable children. Therefore, when children receive vaccines they are not only protecting their own health, but the health of others.

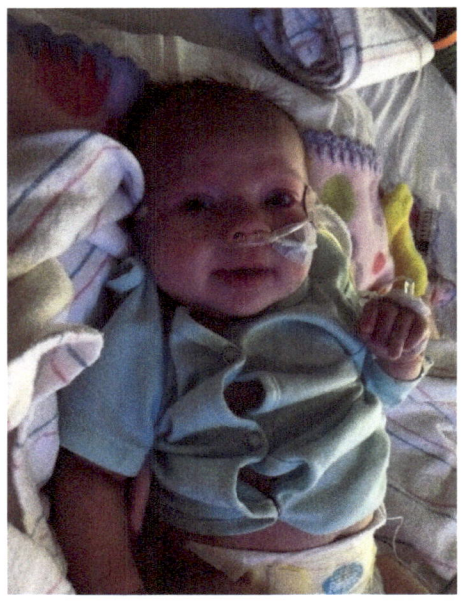

This is Everlee when she was six weeks old.

More information about childhood vaccination can be found at:

www.voicesforvaccines.org

www.vaccineinformation.org

http://vec.chop.edu

Books about vaccination:

Your Baby's Best Shot: Why Vaccines Are
Safe and Save Lives,
by Stacy Mintzer Herlihy and E. Allison Hagood

Baby 411: Clear Answers & Smart Advice For
Your Baby's First Year,
by Denise Fields and Dr. Ari Brown

What to Expect Guide to Immunizations,
by Heidi Murkoff and Sharon Mazel

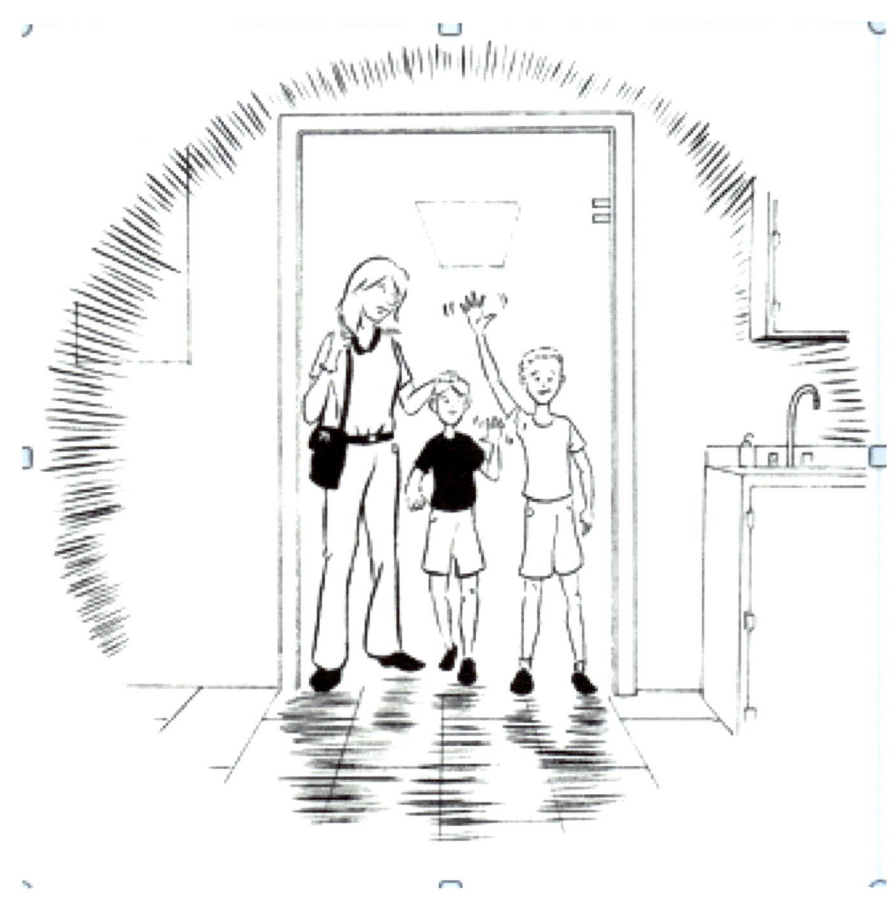

www.ingramcontent.com/pod-product-compliance
Lightning Source LLC
Chambersburg PA
CBHW040317010626
45792CB00023B/1005